Surviving A DiagnosiS

Hope

On the Other Side

By K. A. Bryant

Hope on the Other Side

Hope on the Other Side

Medical Disclaimer

All content found in Surviving A Diagnosis, Hope on the Other Side & The Workbook, including: text, images, audio, or other formats were created for informational purposes only. The Content is not intended to be a substitute for professional medical advice, diagnosis, or treatment. Always seek the advice of your physician or other qualified health provider with any questions you may have regarding a medical condition. Never disregard professional medical advice or delay in seeking it because of something you have read in this book.

If you think you may have a medical emergency, call your doctor, or go to the emergency department. Lakehouse Publishing
L.L.C. does not recommend or endorse any specific tests, medical facilities, physicians, products, procedures, opinions, or other information that may be mentioned in the Surviving A Diagnosis book. Reliance on any information provided by this content is solely at your own risk.

The names of characters have been changed. Any similarities are purely coincidental.

Published by LAKEHOUSE PUBLISHING L.L.C. © 2019

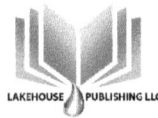

Copyright © 2019 Surviving A DiagnosiS

Hope On the Other Side

ISBN: 978-1-7347112-3-3/ Amz: ISBN: 979-8-6480048-1-8/ 9798664202380 ISBN: 978-1-7347112-4-0

Thank you for choosing this book.
Get more books by joining the
K. A. BRYANT mailing list on
kabryant.com.

Hope on the Other Side

To all those

Surviving a diagnosis.

May you never lose
Hope.

Hope on the Other Side

Preface

Janice Smith crosses an invisible bridge as she sits in the doctor's chair listening to words that she never thought she would hear. The bridge leads her from her familiar world of carefree good health across to the unfamiliar world of terminal illness. What she doesn't know is that there is hope on the other side.

On the way to her car, the overstuffed folder filled with random papers explaining her medical condition slips from her hand. On her knees, teary eyed, she gathers them into a disordered pile and shoves them into the car door. At home, confused and saddened, she flips through them for hours just before bed and realizes that they only address the logistical side of her condition but leave her day-to-day living a mystery.

She searches the papers but can't find the missing piece to her puzzle. She can't find it because half of it is in your hand. "Surviving A Diagnosis, Hope on the Other Side" is the true story account of her life. The other half of the missing piece is in The Workbook. "Surviving A Diagnosis, Hope on the Other Side & The Workbook is a combination of this book and The Workbook so you will be getting two books in one. I encourage you to get it. It's a full color paperback you will use daily."

Definition of survive (verb):
1: to remain alive or in existence: live on
2: to continue to function or prosper despite

You are a survivor. This book will encourage and empower you. "The Workbook" gives you the tools you will need to survive a diagnosis day-to-day. If you are caring for a loved one with a diagnosis, this book will be a valuable guide to help them get through it and it will make caring for them easier.

There is a symptom log, grocery list, do's and don'ts and more. It also has advice for setting up your healing-home space. There are tips for pre-treatment and post-treatment issues regardless of your diagnosis.

If you have a common cold, this book is probably not for you. It is ideal for people who have chronic long-term illnesses and even terminal illnesses. Sometimes, we can't control what happens, but we can control what we believe while it's happening.

Healing, mentally, physically and spiritually is very important to me. "K-Today" is dedicated to this. There is an online course for "Surviving A Diagnosis" that goes deeper into these topics with audio and video so move at your own pace. Understanding that sometimes, you may not feel up to sitting up at a computer and engaging, there is an exclusive podcast on "Live Your Life With Kay" channel via YouTube. You can find it all on https://liveyourlifewithkay.com.

God desires us to be whole. I Thessalonians 5:23;

"And the very God of peace sanctify you wholly; and I pray God your whole spirit and soul body be preserved blameless unto the coming of our Lord Jesus Christ."

CHAPTER ONE

Present Day... Waiting

Still waiting. The nurse said the results would be ready today and they've always called with test results early in the morning. But it's already 11:30 and nothing. The phone only rang once. My mother, who called to share her morning inspirational scripture. I look forward to those perhaps more than she knows. That, and a cup of coffee in my breakfast nook beside the window showered by the morning Texas sun. I enjoy the scriptures, but I think it's her voice that I look forward to hearing most of all. Before this occurred, I planned to run, like my father. He taught me life lessons on that track; but his ability to honor commitment, despite circumstances, was his biggest unspoken lesson learned.

Folding clothes is therapeutic. Creating perfect department-store stacks of folded fresh smelling clothes keeps my hands busy and my mind occupied. Aligning the corners, I smooth the soft material. The smell of the fabric softener fills the house and that ominous pile decreases.

It's funny how even after one has a baby, the stomach and organs take time to settle back into place. Until they do, I will look four months pregnant. It never bothered me to be mistaken for being pregnant, when I was pregnant. Afterward, it's just a bold reminder that I must do some crunches.

Why hasn't she called yet? This is torturous. This time, not even the loud enthusiastic preaching on the television can stop my mind from slipping into worry. Focus, focus. It's my favorite video of the summer tent church service.

Every year, the church set up an enormous tent in one of the most dangerous parks in Queens, New York. Why go outside in a dangerous park in the heat when we have a perfectly good edifice? This question was answered at the end of the first service.

Surprise!

To Do List

- ☑ Laundry
- ☐ Wash the dog
- ☐ Grocery Shopping
- ☐ O. B. Appointment
- ☐ Call Mom

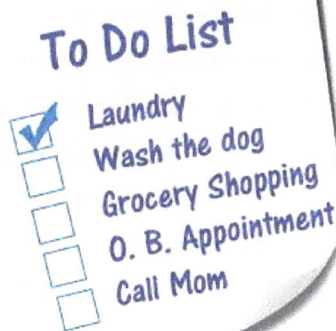

I should start at the top. Two months ago, a grand business plan was brewing in the back of my mind and we were at the precipice of a fresh start. New house, new State, why not? I never could sit still for long. It's just not in my genes. This vision was clear, and I couldn't wait to discuss it with Charles. I had the time-line planned and details set. Then, walking out of the kitchen one night, I paused mid-step, looked at Charles and ran to the bathroom and threw up. You guessed it. It was not the flu. I was expecting. Instant joy.

My pregnancies were beautiful. Back aches and swollen feet all came with the package, and that was expected. However, throughout this pregnancy I felt no back pain, no further nausea, and didn't feel the weight of my baby bump at all. Charles, however, had nausea and two trips to the emergency room for excruciating lower back pain in the middle of the night. A battery of test found nothing and at the end, an experienced nurse comically told him 'you are carrying her pregnancy'.

That was a lot to carry because I was huge. My baby bump was more like a mountain. I can smile about it now, holding up tiny baby clothes, but I was so large that when people saw me, they cringed. I've heard; 'That's got to hurt' more times than I care to mention. The funny thing was, all the weight was in my stomach. So, I waddled like a swollen duck.

I forgot what it felt like to sleep on my stomach and promised myself that as soon as I delivered; I wanted two things. First, a strong cup of coffee and the second, to sleep on my stomach for the rest of my life.

The days passed quickly, and I had a perfect routine. My to-do list was always full. I rose early, went through my morning routine and saw Charles out the door off to work while the Texas sun was just getting warmed-up. It was yet to unleash its full fury over the brick homes in our neighborhood. Houston was fresh territory for us, but we were unintimidated about starting over here. It felt more like an adventure. There is something about being a native New Yorker that drilled strength into me little by little, starting from the first time you ride your tricycle down your driveway. A deep breath and I glance at the framed photos on the mantle, a reflection of our past years.

However, it wasn't the New York grit that gave me the strength to deal with what was coming next. It couldn't. This needed something more. To negate a force, it requires an equal or greater force. This required strength from a deeper level. A spiritual level. To survive what was coming next, I needed power in the core of my being.

Go Away!

One morning I was spotting. Never the word a seven-month pregnant woman wants to say. It was the first telltale sign that something was wrong. Was I dilating? Who knows? Waiting for the doctor to return with her instructions was very uncomfortable. The chairs in examination rooms lack all forms of comfort.

My doctor is focused yet friendly. Her personality suit mine perfectly. She was not a chatty person. She came to the point quickly. She walks into the examination room with the nurse with papers in her hand and says one routine-changing word.

"Bed rest. I want you on bed-rest for the rest of your pregnancy. We'll run some additional tests too." Said the doctor.

That was the verdict so there I lay, early in the morning watching Charles get dressed for work and the morning sun rising without me. He gave me a kiss and had a funny smirk on his face, knowing that I was not likely to stay in the bed. He knows me very well. I heard the backdoor lock behind him and before the car rolled out of the driveway; I was out of bed.

That day, I found a million reasons to get out of bed until I gathered all the things I needed. I placed them at arms-reach to make bed rest possible for me. I had a full desk set up on the side of the bed, fax machine, laptop computer, telephone and notebooks. The business plan was buzzing around in my head and I wanted to have every detail together to present to Charles when he got home. Besides, it wasn't my first time on bed rest. I knew how this went. Feet up, drink lots of water and before I know it, I will have the all clear. The day went quickly, and I heard Charles's keys clinking at the backdoor.

"Really?" said Charles, standing in the bedroom doorway.

I could smell the delicious aroma coming from the bags in his hands. His tie loosened and a smirk on his face. He didn't look surprised at all. The dog, my accomplice, curled at my feet in a white puffy ball, lifted his head and looked at Charles as if he were pleading his case.

"Oh, you bought dinner. How wonderful." I said.

"Don't change the subject." He shook his head.

He placed the bags on the foot of the bed and put his finger up then disappeared into the family room with our other children giggling and running behind him. I re-adjusted my weight and sat up tall. I already had my 'to do' lists written out for tomorrow. With the new business outline laid out, there was an excitement in the air about the baby coming.

It's funny sitting here now, folding the same baby clothes that I had helplessly saw sitting in their bags on the rocking chair just months ago. I missed doing laundry from that day. There were so many exciting things happening and I couldn't wait to get back on my feet.

"Push guys." I heard Charles say from the family room.

Then the fifty-five-inch television on its platform came rolling head first into the bedroom. It was immense.

"What!" I laughed in shock.

The kids giggled and pushed beside him with a broad smile on their faces. He rolled up his sleeves to connect the wiring. I can still recall when he purchased it in New York. We worked together in our own business for over a decade until one Saturday morning during prayer, the Lord laid it on our hearts to move. We planned to call a real estate agent first thing on Monday morning.

Logistically, it made no sense. The business was successful and growing. But God said it was time to move. The year, 2016, and that summer was hot, but we couldn't feel it at all. The air conditioner in the house ran night and day. That Monday morning at seven-thirty, the phone rang. It was someone saying that they were in prayer that morning and God put it in their heart to call Charles. They didn't know exactly why God told them to call. They had been praying for guidance because they were trying to move. They thought perhaps that Charles had some advice on moving that would be helpful for them.

Charles spoke with them and learned that they were house hunting for almost a year. They were ready to purchase with a pre-approval already in hand. The amazing thing about this was the region they were looking for a home in. They were looking to purchase a few blocks away from us.

We set an appointment for them to see the house on Wednesday. We toured them through the house, then we all sat and talked for hours. They didn't leave until after eleven o'clock at night. They wanted the house.

On Thursday morning, lawyers were contacted, and the rest was history. Our home was not put on the real estate market. We never held a showing. We never even used a real estate agent. God knew both of our circumstances, and everything worked out for the best for all of us.

However, biggest miracle was yet to come. Months later, the worst housing market crash since the great depression hit the United States. That house sold just before it happened, and because of when we sold, we received the true value of our house. The reason for our move, which would never have happened if God didn't guide us to sell, was coming up.

Nibbling on the best hot honey glazed rolls I've ever tasted. Charles served the children on paper plates and they sat cross-legged, chewing away between giggles. Charles sat bed beside me on the bed enjoying tender roast beef, mashed potatoes and buttery corn. I wriggled my way out of the bed with Charles's help.

"Bathroom."

It was then that I saw something I pray no pregnant woman will ever see. More blood. Not just spotting. Far more than spotting. Concerned, but knowing I didn't really honor the bed rest order, I thought it would resolve itself. Tomorrow, I would have true bed rest. Knowing this wasn't normal, I pulled myself together and stepped out of the bathroom.

"I need to call the doctor." I said.

We were concerned but our faith was strong.

"Flat on your back, bed rest." The doctor said. I listened intently. "All day. Only get up to go to the bathroom. I'm sending you a nurse, a monitor, and blood pressure monitor linked to a center. Keep them on all day and night. Okay?"

Her tone, flat. I knew this was serious. I also knew that it wasn't unusual to deliver in the seventh month. With today's technology, it wouldn't be detrimental to the baby. But that was not what any of us wanted. 'Full term, Lord', that was my prayer and belief.

Bed Rest

Horizontal bed rest meant that I would lie on my left side for a great deal of time. Lying flat on my back was not an option. If I laid on my right side, my arm or leg fell asleep quickly. Charles brought me about four pillows, yet I was uncomfortable. I often heard our pastor say that sometimes, when you're ready to bring forth a big blessing, things become uncomfortable.

The wires from the monitor wrapped around my stomach and connected to a gray machine that beeped softly beside the bed. I was grateful for the television in the bedroom. It helped pass the time along with my fluffy companion who sat faithfully beside the bed facing the doorway. He was always on guard. I noticed that his little puppy character changed. He was somber. His mood matched mine. He was a great comfort, especially with the children being in school. He listened to all of my corny jokes and never walked away once. It was as if he knew something was wrong and instinctively did what a good friend would, stay right by my side.

Questions without answers were already swarming in my head. I quelled them with simple answers such as, 'it's just because of my age' and 'this too shall pass'. It's funny, but I recalled quoting scriptures and my faith was strong. I believed that it was just a test. I believed that this would pass. Each appointment, I expected that it would be the appointment that the doctor would give me pleasant news that would erase the need for me to wake up pulling on my faith.

Weeks passed and my body was feeling the effect of carrying the baby along with tiredness from laying all day. Like most pregnant woman at the end of the third trimester, I couldn't sleep because the bold movement of a full-term baby turning woke me frequently during the night. It exhausted me inside and out. Things transformed in a short amount of time.

CHAPTER TWO

In the Middle

To Do List

- [ ] O.B. Appointment
- [ ] Read
- [x] Review business plan
- [ ] Call Mom

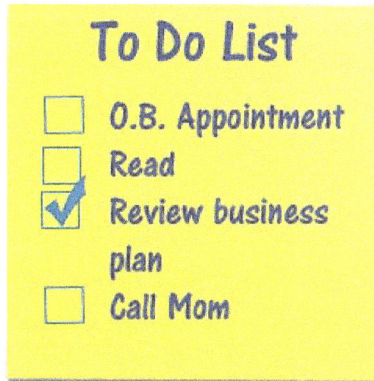

Praying has been a part of my life since I gave my life to Christ at nineteen. However, I have never had to pray for good health. No hospital stays or medical issues other than a common cold. I focused on eating healthy and exercising. The only long-term physical issue I have ever dealt with was trying to lose weight. But this circumstance put me into a more serious prayer-place. I needed to pray every morning just to function. We love God, pray, spent most of our time in church. Surely, if anyone would come out with a blessed testimony, it would be me. I didn't think this out of arrogance. No. I did not believe I deserved it somehow by works, I knew better than that. Trials come, that's a part of life, but God always saw us through. Why should this time be any different?

As promised, the doctor ran a battery of tests. When the results came in, I called the office as usual to get them, but was told that the doctor wanted to give me the results in person. That was odd. Charles thought it peculiar, yet, like me, we expected the best. He took off from work; we picked the kids up from school and headed to the doctor's office with juice boxes and snacks. He parked the car on the side of the office, put a show on in the truck for the children as I went in. I sat in the doctor's office on the examination table. The door closed and the crinkly paper rustled with my every wiggle. My first indication that something was definitely wrong was when the nurse came in.

"Follow me, please." She said holding out her hand.

Silent, she helped me down from the table and I notice her continence. She was with me, but not *with* me. I knew her well. After nine-months of jokes and small talk, she behaved like a stranger. She said nothing. She led me down the hall to the doctor's office and opened the door. Facing me was a wall of windows and to my surprise, our truck parked right there alongside the office.

I take a seat and she told me the doctor would be in soon. She left the office door open halfway. I saw Charles seated behind the wheel and waved at him, but the three o'clock Texas sun made it impossible for him to see beyond the glare on the office building glass. He looked directly in my direction for a moment. I waved vigorously, but his expression showed he didn't see me at all. An eerie feeling shot through me. The feeling of being present but not acknowledged as a complete person. The feeling of being present, but not here. Strangely, that is how I felt with the nurse. Something changed and I didn't know what it was and couldn't explain it. I felt as if I was on the other side of the glass and the glare of something kept her from seeing me.

Time dragged, waiting for the doctor to come into the room. I read every diploma, certificate, award and news article that hung on her office wall behind her desk. Finally, the door opened, and the doctor entered with papers in her hand. She yelled a few orders to a nurse, then closed the door behind her. No formalities, she jumped straight to the point. I expected nothing less.

"Sorry for the wait." She leaned on the desk in front of me. "I had them double check the results and re-run the labs." She tilted her head compassionately. I took a deep breath, trying to imagine what it could be. The baby was moving normally. We had a heart-beat and the sonogram looked great. Then she spoke. "It's cancer."

The word was rubber. It bounced off of me like a ball. It just didn't stick. It couldn't. I was a Christian. A believer, a faith-filled tither, a go big or go home praise and worshiper. Nope. Not receiving it. Not today or ever. She kept talking. I heard her words as a faint murmur, I can't recall what her exact words. Then, as if a veil lifted, a small pick dug in.

"If these results are right, Janice, it is advanced." She lifts a page. "We don't have time to waste. It means... you have about... two years to live." The doctor glues her eyes on mine.

Not having digested what she said, I just stared at her emotionless. My mind didn't fathom those words being said to me. Looking back, I may have been in some in informational shock. I felt as if she was talking to someone who was standing in my body, not me I recalled wondering if this is what having strong faith made you feel when you got terrible news. If so, I liked it. One question rolled to the front of my mind and out of my mouth.

"How does this affect the baby?" I ask.

"I will be honest with you, I'm not an oncologist so I'm not the best person to deal with this. M. D. Anderson Cancer Center is where you need to be. It's downtown in the Medical District." She pulled a pen from her pocket and scribbled on a thick notepad on her desk, tears the page off and handed me the paper. "This is what I want you to do. Go there." I glanced at the paper. It's an address. "Whatever they tell you to do, just do it. They know what they're talking about. They are the best in the world." She helped me stand and we walked toward the door.

When she opened her office door and I was unprepared for what was in front of me. Every eye in the office was on me. The entire staff already knew. They were searching my face for a reaction. These were women I saw regularly for months. They knew me. Exchanged pleasantries with me and what I saw next was brutal. They bowed their heads at their desks as if Janice was already dead. Cancer took the center stage. They didn't say a word. Did *it* have a stronger presence than I? A bolder personality capable of eradicating my very being?

"Here," the doctor took a package from a nurse and handed it to me, "This is your entire medical record. Give this to them. Can you go now?"

"Yes... I guess." Alarmed at her urgency.

"Good, I'll call ahead. They will run their own tests." She walked me to the outer office door. It felt as if she wanted to get rid of me. An awful feeling.

As soon as I walked out of the office door, I looked at Charles through the windshield. I saw him pause as our eyes locked. He knew by my expression that something wasn't right. I didn't want to spread this news to him. I didn't want to put on his shoulders, what now laid on mine, but I had no choice.

Lots of hands

He held my hand firm enough to let me know he was there, but gentle enough to not crack anything. That's what we did all the way downtown that day, and every time afterward when we drove to an appointment in M. D. Anderson. Hands. Lots of holding hands. It was just what I needed. I needed to feel that I wasn't alone and not invisible. But even with his support, a sinking feeling set in every moment it got a chance. I believe that God never gives one more than they can bear. He knew I couldn't bear this alone.

We sat so close on the couch during date night, you couldn't squeeze a pin between us. We watched movies and ate popcorn. The movies took me to an unfamiliar place. They pulled me into a world where there was no cold reality of the unknown. It was action, fun and adventure.

One night, in particular, I barely saw the movie. Instead, I watched the children sitting beside us on the sofa, eyes wide on a cartoon movie we selected for them and just felt the warmth of his hand. Then an uninvited thought crept into my mind.

What if I weren't here? How much pressure would that put on Charles? I just assumed I would always be here to see them grow up. I assumed tomorrow would always be there and that I had millions of Christmas' to see. Uncountable birthdays and holidays to decorate for. I never considered not being able to plant my garden in spring.

Charles and I even talked about what it would be like to become grandparents and travel the world. It couldn't be that everything I believed I would do, couldn't be accomplished. I felt promises trying to slip away. Until now, I never saw time as something that was being spent. A new battle even greater than cancer had begun. The battle to hold on to hope, on the other side.

I never focused on the aspect of healthy or unhealthy. When the most you have ever faced has been a common cold, it was easy to take health for granted. I felt the other side becoming a strong reality little by little. It was time to put to work everything I learned in church. Gratitude for having a Christian foundation filled me every morning that I saw the sun. It was now that I saw life in 'time'.

Before, I overlooked time. It got lost amid thinking about what's for dinner tomorrow or lost in the next science project. Invincibility diminished. Though I said it many times, I now understood that my life was NOT in *my* hands. When I declared "Lord, have your way," honestly, I never considered that 'His way' would be anything like this. I realized I didn't grasp what I was saying. Life and death are in the power of the tongue. (Proverbs 8:21).

Hope on the Other Side

CHAPTER THREE

Blind Date

To Do List

- ☑ 8am MRI
- ☐ 8:30 CT Scan
- ☐ 9:30 PET Scan
- ☐ 10:00 Blood Work
- ☐ 11:00 Radiologist
- ☐ 12:00 Specialist

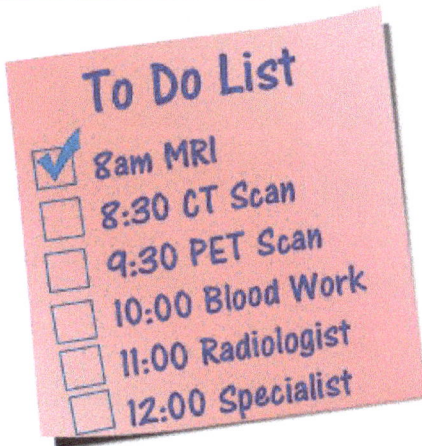

These memories are bitter, but it seems appropriate that they flood into my mind now, waiting for the test results. The beginning of the journey was the worst. Almost finished folding this load of laundry, the buzz of the dryer's timer lets me know that the next load is ready. I exhale and lean back on the sofa, close my eyes and feel the warmth of the sun lay on my face. The curtain is parted; the yard is visible. I know that the grass is deep green and that the roses are bright yellow, but they don't appear to be. They haven't for a while now.

Colors are dull, muted. Living in a gray world is not pleasant. The funny thing is, I noticed this dulling of color mostly with the color green and all variations of it. Also, my distinction between textures changed. Things seem to fall within soft or rough. Life feels surreal. The funny thing is, I can't recall the exact day these changes crept in.

Perhaps that is why I enjoy folding the soft clothes. I feel them; I smell them, and it is comforting. I spoke with my doctor about this, and I expected an elaborate medical or technical reply. But it wasn't. She said that she has had several patients who experienced a difference in how colors appear to them while going through treatment, although their cancer didn't involve their brain. She called it 'cancer on the brain'.

She also said that it was temporary, and most patients stated their perception returned to normal post-treatment. Breathless, weak and the fragility of this body is sobering. This is unlike anything I ever experienced.

Unable to raise my hands above my head, combing my hair is a chore and takes three times as long as it did before. Even lying in bed, I breathe heavily as if I just ran around a track full-speed. I have yet to see the color return to my life.

A small pile of shirts falls from the sofa. Exhaling, I lean forward and pick them up. My hand brushes a piece of paper sticking out from beneath the sofa. It is a sticky note of one of my old 'to do' lists. The sting of fresh tears form in my eyes and the thought that life may never be as simplistic as it once was, fills my mind. The memory of the day my 'to do' list changed will stay with me forever.

I recalled when I sat at the kitchen desk, pen in hand, and scrawled out an ominous to-do list. Laundry was no longer my most challenging thing to do for the day. Charles and I still I believed that this was a wrong diagnosis or that God would perform an instant healing miracle. Eager, we left for M. D. Anderson to start the battery of tests, believing their results would show that there was no cancer in my body.

It was easy to envision myself shouting for joy and spreading my testimony of how God healed me and spared me from having to undergo the feigned treatment. I pictured the doctors comparing the two test results and shaking their heads in disbelief, baffled at the undeniable miracle they would say, "How is this possible?" I would reply, "God is real". If this were my testimony, the book would probably end here. However, what came of it was awe-inspiring. We trekked on, from one appointment to the other. It was a long and exhausting day.

The wonderful thing about M. D. Anderson in Houston, Texas was that it designed and run with the patient's comfort in mind. Aesthetically, uncluttered, with expansive halls and minimalist signs to guide but not intimidate.

All testing centers were within the facility. We felt relieved about not having to drive across town to various labs. They had a scheduling strategy that I understood by my last appointment of the day. I had expected to see my assigned physician first. I didn't. They scheduled me to see her last.

Still very pregnant, I waddled through the corridors with Charles. When we moved from New York and ended up in Houston, we had no idea that the house we would purchase would be forty-five minutes from M. D.

Anderson. We didn't even know about M. D. Anderson and never thought we would need it. But God knew. We went from waiting room to waiting room. Ate lunch in their dining hall, then continued with our appointments. Optimistic, we took it in stride, believing that this would be our first and only visit to M. D. Anderson Cancer Center.

I saw some things I never saw before and would not have seen had this circumstance not come about. I saw cancer patients in wheelchairs covered in warm blankets. Some people wore medical masks. Some people had no hair. Some had family with them, but some wondered the halls wide-eyed and alone until one of M. D. Anderson's volunteers that dot the facility halls offered help.

Hands clasped behind their backs, volunteers stood in soft blue vests loaded with buttons and badges. Cancer survivors themselves, they offered directions, information, and even walked patients to their destination with a compassion only earned from having gone through it themselves. The most important thing they offered was that smile. That unforgettable smile reminding you, they 'saw you'. Not cancer, they saw you. I appreciated that smile more than they may ever know.

Finally, we got through the battery of tests and we were waiting to see my doctor. The idea behind the scheduling was that by the time a patient saw their doctor, which was the last appointment, their test results were in and the doctor could give them to the patient. Charles and I prayed silently as we waited for our turn. The funny thing was that we prayed for everyone else. We truly believed my healing was just moments away. Then they called my name.

"Janice Smith." Said the nurse.

It was like walking into something blind. An unwanted blind date. We never experienced this before. The doctor and nurse were in the room with Charles and I.

I sat on the examination table and Charles sat in a chair holding my purse on his lap. She tapped the tablet in her hand that had my full medical chart and test results on it. Then she told us the results. My heart was pounding with excitement. My lips curled upward in the corner, holding back a long-awaited smile. I longed to hear confirming words. Words that would release me from the grip of turmoil that was trying to take place in my heart.

Not Today

"No, they must be wrong." I said to her.

Charles shook his head 'no' slightly.

"I'm afraid there is no mistake."

I paused inside and out. Time seemed to stand still. I battled with accepting this as my new reality. I felt fine physically. This didn't make accepting their words any easier. I had no 'illness' symptoms. No pain anywhere. If it were not for blood tests, this would not even have been found.

There were two options before me. One, deny the diagnosis and walk out touting that I believe God wouldn't do this to me. Two, stay and listen to what they had to say and accept a treatment plan. The choice was mine. I had a strong faith and so did Charles. God did miraculous

32

healing miracles all the time, so it stood to reason that I could be a candidate. Knowing the Word of God became so significant right at that moment. I felt myself lean on God in an another way. Our pastor always said that there was a fine line between faith and foolishness. He taught us that he who is whole need not a physician.

"But when Jesus heard that, he said unto them, They that be whole need not a physician, but they that are sick." (KJV) Matthew 9:12.

Would it be faith or foolishness to walk away? Or can I have faith in the treatment plan being of God? In an instant, with all eyes on me, these thoughts ran through my mind. I believed that:

"The steps of a good man are ordered by the Lord: and he delighteth in his way." (KJV) Psalm 37:23.

Was it possible that of all places on the earth that God could have moved to, He sent us here for this very reason? Did he move us here so I could have access to the best medical treatment in the world? Suddenly, I believed so. Thus, I took a deep breath and replied.

"So, what do you suggest?" I asked.

"First, you're in the right place. I have already contacted our radiology department and you will meet with one of our top experts in this area. She'll tell you your options. If you're ready, you can go straight there. The sooner you see her, the better." Said the doctor, pleased to see my receptiveness.

A mix of feelings fell in the pot. First, disbelief. We left the office and were silent for a moment. Then, Charles spoke positive words and proclaimed and decreed that God will perform a miracle in this. Sometimes miracles happen immediately, and sometimes God walks you through them. We walked to the radiologist's office and spoke to her for over forty-five minutes. I asked every question I could think of. I was skeptical. But, by the end of the appointment, it was clear that this would not be a quick-fast miracle, not today. Not for me. From her account, the journey was a long one and only held the possibility of 'cure'. That's a word you don't hear often about cancer.

"You said, 'cured'?" I asked.

"This treatment is aggressive." She said. Her legs crossed wearing a long crisp white lab coat. "The human body can only endure it once in its lifetime. It must be done correctly the first time. Janice, we only get one shot at this. Even with everything done precisely, I will be honest with you, there is still no guarantee it will work." She uncrossed her legs, rested her elbows on her knees, and leaned in toward me. "You have a special circumstance. You see, cells reproduce faster in pregnancy. All cells. It's the nature of the body forming a baby. Unfortunately, the same is true for cancer cells. The cancer is not in your lymph nodes. That means it is only in the tumor. The more time goes by, the more it can spread. Once it hits the lymph nodes, containing it is difficult if not impossible." She crossed her legs again and her facial expression intensified with a deep breath.

"I'm afraid you have a choice to make. If we wait until the baby is born, we have no guarantee that it will not spread to the lymph nodes before we start the treatment. You have three weeks left to delivery and with cancer, three weeks is a long time. However, if we take this aggressive action now, well, we also can't guarantee what repercussions it may have on the baby. I'm sorry, there is no simple answer here." Her eyes shift from Charles's to mine, then back again. "You two have allot to think about, but you have little time to do it."

"Would you give us a moment?" Charles asked.

She left the room and we had a conversation that didn't lead to an immediate answer. There was so much to consider, and questions came up in our conversation. When she returned, we asked more questions.

"What does this treatment entail?" I asked.

"Radiation, chemotherapy and then a three-day Hospital stay of round-the-clock radiation. We hit that tumor with everything we can."

"Why can't we just cut it out?"

She adjusted her lab coat and uncrossed her legs. She was pleasant and seemed glad to hear our questions. Later, she told me she was always happy to see patients engaged in their treatment plan and asking questions. It was the start of an informed and engaged patient.

"Cancer functions on a cellular level. Surgery is not as effective for your stage as radiation and chemotherapy. Using surgery, there is still a high likelihood of it returning."

The more we listened, the more we saw the face of what we were dealing with. On our way to the car, a book-sized folder stacked with papers handed me by each person in my health team slipped. They scattered on the floor, lifted by the hot wind. I almost wished the wind blew them so far from my world that I would never see them again. On bended knee, we scooped them together. My eye caught sight of the titles. "The Side Effects of Chemotherapy", "Healthy Eating", "Side Effects of Radiation".

Later, at home, I thumbed through them. There contents were terrifying. Silent, tired and bursting with information, we did what came natural to us. We held hands and prayed. If that's all we did that day, it would have been plenty.

Redefined

Something sat on me that night. A sobering reality that I had to face this. I praised, but it was still there. I prayed, but it didn't go away. It redefined my life. This was supposed to be a fleeting testimony that inspired others. But now, it was here every morning I woke. The next day I took my prenatal vitamin and ate breakfast. Then the questions flowed.

How did this slip in? Was there something I did wrong? How did this get in under the prayer radar? I am a planner. My parents taught me to be forward thinking and to plan to prevent things ever since I was a child. This was something I couldn't plan for. This was beyond my control on all levels. There was one thing left to do, my homework. I needed to know for certain that this was the best treatment plan for me.

My laptop was occasionally used to indulge my bursts of curiosity for information, but this was the biggest work-over I ever gave it. I looked at everything. In college, studying Psychology, I read case studies, so medical jargon didn't intimidate me. I read case studies about cancer treatments performed all around the world and matched it with the information the radiologist gave us and found everything she said to be true. I researched the studies done on the prescribed chemotherapy drug and its effectiveness compared to others. My conclusion, everything I was told at M. D. Anderson was true.

If we, and I say we because Charles and I went through this together, did not do the treatment, my life expectancy was two-and-a half years at the most. I prayed and cried and thought. What hit home hard was the list of side-effects of chemotherapy. It was three pages long. It was the most terrifying thing I ever read. Prior, my greatest challenge was whether to get highlights this summer. This decision was overwhelming.

I thought that losing hair was the worst of it. That was what I always associated cancer with. Until today, cancer was someone else's illness. My ignorance in this area showed me what a carefree lifestyle I lived just by being able to enjoy good health. We had no time to waste. We decided.

I knew that God gave us this baby for a reason and that risking its life was not an option for me. The baby deserved every opportunity to come into this world as perfect as God created it to be. And it was perfectly healthy. I told the doctor my decision to wait on treatment and she reiterated the possible consequences and asked me if I was certain. I told her I was sure.

Charles' support was priceless at this critical point. Being on one accord and respecting one another's feelings was crucial. She said that two weeks after delivery she would re-test me to see if the tumor grew or if the cancer got into my lymph nodes. If, after we had the baby, they found if cancer to be in my lymph nodes, she would have to reassess my treatment plan and the options. The prognosis would change.

Until then, the next two weeks would be normal for me. I would eat what I craved and carry on normally until the delivery. I played with my children, did laundry and just felt normal. I didn't want to tell people that I had something that would make them categorize me and pity me or even look at me as if I were dying. Normalcy. That's what I wanted.

In a weak moment, I called my obstetrician and asked her to do the surgery. Radiation and chemotherapy terrified me. If she said yes, I was going through with it. Then I could throw those wretched side effects sheets away and never go back to M. D. Anderson. Brilliant, right? No.

I tried so hard to get the memory of M. D. Anderson out of my mind. The blank expressions on the faces of people seated in those waiting rooms. Fear knows no age, race or financial status. Helplessness overwhelmed some people and others, hopelessness. I saw it on the young, the old, the middle-aged, on women and men.

There were people being pushed in wheelchairs that looked as if they wanted to stand and push their own chair. They had a flicker of life, will to live and fight burning deep inside of them.

Charles and I met people from all over the world who flew to Houston just to go to M. D. Anderson for treatment. In those elevators we weren't Americans, Italians or British. We were people. Just people fighting for a chance to live. I didn't feel strong enough to face that again. I needed my life back and surgery was comprehensible to me. Chemotherapy and radiation were not.

"Can you remove it?" I asked the doctor.

"Yes, technically, I can do the surgery but... what did M. D. Anderson say?" the doctor asked.

"They suggested radiation and chemo. But I trust you. I'll let you do the surgery." I said fighting back tears.

"Janice, I'll be honest with you. If that's what M. D. Anderson recommended, then surgery's not the best thing for you. If I were you. I would do what they said."

Our call ended with me in agreement to follow M. D. Anderson's treatment plan. When a doctor that could get paid allot of money to do a surgery says no, one must re-consider. Okay, Lord. God's answer was obvious.

This tries relationships. It wasn't a cold or even the flu. It will bring out the best in a relationship or show it the worst in it. Before it is all over, at the very least, one knows exactly what they are married to.

Charles and I got closer. I looked into his eyes and could tell when he was physically tired yet, he never complained. For the time being, everything felt normal. We shopped and lived and enjoyed every day. Life felt normal for the next few weeks.

The baby was born perfectly healthy. However, the delivery didn't have the suspense typical of a baby delivery. We weren't sitting around waiting for the water to break. The delivery was completely planned. The doctor set the date for a weekday to ensure that specialists were on duty. It went smoothly despite the circumstances.

Two weeks later, I re-tested at M. D. Anderson to see if the size of the tumor changed or if the cancer spread to the lymph nodes. The results brought me to my knees the moment I got into my prayer closet.

There was no change. It didn't grow or spread at all. We could proceed with the original treatment plan. We gave God all the glory and asked for strength to face what lay ahead. The doctor was surprised that it didn't change at all. Although the big testimony of the cancer being gone completely didn't happen, I learned to see the other miracles that were clear. That we even lived near the facility. That God moved us when he did and to where he did. Then, that the cancer would not even have been found if it were not for the pregnancy, was a miracle. It's easy to miss those blessings in the absence of the expected larger one.

Hope on the Other Side

CHAPTER FOUR

Here We Go!

To Do List

☑ 5:00 am Wake Up

☐ 7:00 am Radiation
treatment #1

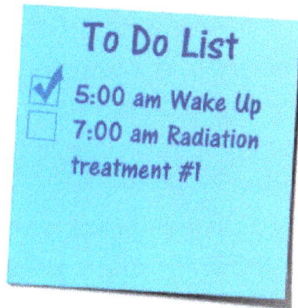

Power, under control, in measured doses isn't destructive. Everything I have ever heard about radiation was terrifying. I could only think of nuclear explosions and every horrifying image that followed one. I realized that this radiation treatment was power under control. The commute to the hospital was longer than the ten second treatment.

In the waiting room, I noticed that most of the women who were also waiting for their treatment wore wigs.

Beautiful wigs. Charles and I agreed that I would wear my long hair up in sensitivity to other women who may have lost their hair.

Some were dressed for work. Some didn't even look like patients. They were working while they waited, productive and vibrant. They seemed as if this was just something they had to do on the way to their other appointments. That confused me because I thought all cancer patients were incapacitated because of the illness.

I also learned that what incapacitated them was usually not the illness. It was the aggressiveness of the radiation and chemotherapy treatment. Cancer cells are aggressive, and we must meet them with an aggressive treatment. Unfortunately, those things also attack the good cells that help fight infection and grow hair, fingernails, taste buds and so forth. This was my simpleton way of understanding it. Through every treatment, I prayed, and I always prayed the same thing:

"Lord, you guide the beam. Let it go where it's supposed to and do what it's supposed to do. You are the great physician and I am in *your* hands."

With that, I heard the tech instruct me to hold my breath and the machine beeped after ten seconds. The radiation machine was intimidating. A remarkable piece of machinery. After a few treatments, I got the sensation of an expansion in my spine. Toward my last few treatments, I was afraid I would hear a pop and something would burst in my back, but it never happened.

Exhaustion. That is the only word to describe what I felt afterward. A tiredness unlike any other. I was breathless just walking three to five steps and had no strength.

To brush my teeth, I had to put the toothpaste on the cabinet and drop my fist on it to get the toothpaste to squirt out. For someone accustomed to being very independent, this was a tough reality to face and there was no specific date to look forward to its ending.

My Song

I was too weak to sing and didn't have the breath for it. I missed it. It is a privilege to sing. Unknowingly, I took the ability to sing for granted. I didn't realize how much I sang either. I was weak inside and out.

Daily life changed on many levels. Warned against hot showers, I resolved myself to taking luke-warm ones because radiation makes the skin at the treatment site very sensitive. I longed to use my scented lotions and perfumes that sat unused on my dressing table. That was another thing I was told not to put on before treatments. Things changed, there was no doubt about that.

Our early morning trip to M. D. Anderson became routine. Every morning we stopped at McDonald's and got two eggs and cheese muffin. I got orange juice and Charles got coffee. We played Gospel music all the way there. Sometimes he sang, and I listened, mouthing the words. I don't know if he realized how soothing his voice was in that moment. He brought joy to a very dismal routine.

Things seemed manageable until my first day of chemotherapy. The chemotherapy drug was known to cause hearing loss and sometimes total deafness in some patients. This rarely posed a threat until the third or fourth treatment. If it didn't happen by then, then I was okay.

In the chemotherapy room, the nurse did everything she could to make me comfortable. The room had glass walls opening to a long hall. There was a curtain in every room that gave you privacy from the room across the hall, but nurses frequently walked the halls looking into every room.

In the room, on a steel pole beside the bed, a small bag hung with a murky fluid. I knew the name of my chemotherapy drug and the dose. I read the bag to make sure it was correct. The nurse connected my chemotherapy treatment into my I. V. I took a deep breath.

Each room had a television with videos to choose from. The nurse helped me select a movie and she popped it into the player and turned on the I.V. drip. Although the room looked like a bedroom, that little bag of murky fluid destroyed its cozy feel.

I tried to focus on the television show, but about halfway into the movie, my vein bulged and raised. Quickly it became discolored and began burning. I called the nurse and she came running in so fast she scared me. Later I learned that if the drug wasn't diluted enough, it could burn through the vein and release the drug into my body and the outcome would not be good. She increased its dilution and it was okay.

I heard a woman crying and moaning and the nurses couldn't stop it. I wanted to leave there and never go back. But then, I felt God in there with me. A comfort, in the room. His strength was made perfect in my weakness. That, I knew.

Present Day

I shuffle back to the sofa and sit down slowly. The phone rings. I grab it eagerly.

"Have you eaten?" asks Charles.

"Coffee and a muffin. You know me." I reply. "I'll call you as soon as the doctor calls. Promise."

We chat briefly then hang up and I can hear the doves in the yard cooing. They cooed when I came home from the hospital that day as well. There cooing takes my mind into that moment we came home after that chemotherapy treatment.

Under Water

I was so glad to leave the hospital that day after chemotherapy. We didn't talk much during the ride home because I felt very weak and breathless. Once at home, three doves walked around in the backyard and cooed.

It was memorable because they didn't fly away as Charles helped me into the house. Charles went to work, and I went straight to bed. Later that evening, we watched a movie, and something changed that still hasn't changed back.

Mid-movie heard a loud high-pitched beep and the hearing in one ear changed. Sound was muffled. I ran my finger over the perimeter of the ear and couldn't hear it. I needed the television louder and read lips to figure out similar words.

Later, the audiologist at M. D. Anderson confirmed that I had some hearing loss of high pitch tones. I was told it was unusual for this to happen after only one session of chemotherapy. My extreme sensitivity to the chemotherapy drug meant that continuing with chemotherapy would mean irreversible and total hearing loss.

My doctor suggested changing my chemotherapy drug however, according to my studies, the one I was taking was the only one with a proven track record with the most favorable result for this treatment. Remember, this was a one-shot deal. All factors had to be at play to maximize the probability of a favorable outcome.

Withdrawing this drug meant reducing the likelihood of success, which increased the possibility of cancer returning. My doctor confirmed my information. I told the doctor that I didn't care if I went deaf. I wanted to live, so I told her I wanted to move forward using it, anyway. She advised against it, citing my age and assuring me that the probability of success is still high, not as high, but still high enough to not risk my hearing for the rest of my life. I took her advice, and we moved forward without the chemotherapy. The stress of 'what if' started to weigh on me immediately. What if it didn't work without the chemotherapy drug? What if this makes it return?

CHAPTER FIVE

The Big Bang

I dove into the Word of God. I listened to it play while I rested. It was a battle to stay encouraged that things would work out well. I constantly made positive affirmations and desperately needed to listen to the Word of God. I liked the weight of the physical Bible in my lap and the crinkling sound when I turned a page.

Now, I just couldn't stay focused. My mind drifted easily, and I found listening to things play enabled me to keep my hands busy. I played preaching tapes and gospel music. When it played, the fear went. When I praised, the glory came. When I worshiped, God let me know I wasn't alone. Praise and worship were and still is a defense against negativity and fear.

I didn't have the breath or strength to praise and worship the way I used to. My praise was now a shaking of my head or tapping of my foot. My worship, a slight lifting of my arms held upward for as long as I could. My consolation knew that God understood.

The most important thing is not *what we give*, it is the sacrifice that we give it out of.

An offering is a sacrifice. For me, those slight movements were sacrifices and God accepted them just as if I sang an entire song at the top of my voice. I came to terms with the fact that my testimony would not be; 'I got a poor doctor's report, and God healed me the next day.' Now, I prayed that living would be my testimony.

It wasn't a question of could God heal me. It was a question of would God heal me. Was it in His perfect will for my life that I live beyond two and a half years? If healing was not in His perfect will, despite my finite understanding, I would have to accept it.

The possibility that I would die, and my story would only be 'she lost her battle with cancer' was a realistic thought. But faith is the substance of things hoped for and the evidence of things not seen.

I didn't want that to be my legacy. The longevity of surviving this diagnosis was now upon me. This was the element that one doesn't face when dealing with a short-term illness. A long-term illness changes the dynamic of life. It pushes the mind to extremes and has a mental affect. The strategy to survive long-term illness differs from handling the common cold. The greatest part of my 'test' was coming on Monday.

I would check into the hospital for a three-day stay and get radiation treatment around the clock for the full three days. There was no hand-holding in this part of the treatment.

Preparation was arduous, and but I settled in my room. Radiation is a scary word, but right here, in this part of my treatment, I learned that faith eliminates fear.

"I'm sorry, Sir. You can't stay." The nurse said to Charles.

"He's fine." I said oblivious to her reasoning.

"No, I'm sorry, but no one can be in here with you when the door closes, and the machine is on. Ever. Not even me." The nurse placed her hand on her chest. It was then that I saw it. Her radiation monitor hanging from a strap around her neck. "You may as well go home, Sir. You can call, but there will be no visitors."

We looked at each other. I don't know what we were thinking, but I never considered that he wouldn't be able to be with me. I had to let him go. I had to release that hand. That hand my fingers studied and knew every inch of. He kissed me goodbye and called me as soon as he got in the car. I told him I'm okay and we made light of the moment but, I felt alone. I felt scared and I wanted him to stay. The nurses bustled about in the room constantly glancing at their watches.

"Janice, are you comfortable?" the nurse asked gently.

"Yes, I'm fine, thank you."

"Here," she handed me the television remote, "it helps take your mind off this. I will monitor you from that." She pointed to a black circular camera mounted just above the television on the wall. "If you are in pain or feel anything unusual, press this," she hands me the nurse's call remote attached to the bed by a thick chord, "and you'll be able to speak to me. I can only stop the treatment for emergencies." She said while she fluffed my pillow.

I still had Charles on the phone so, he heard everything. I almost wish I hung up the phone because I didn't want to give him anything additional to think about.

"Thank you." I said.

"Don't worry," she put her hand gently on my ankle while she walked toward the door, "it will be fine." She said pointing to the camera again.

Then she pulled the door and I noticed the most frightening thing Charles and I overlooked when entering the room. The door was as thick as a bank vault door. It closed behind her slowly, then I heard what sounded like a prison door's bolt shut and a vacuum seal sound. I took a deep breath and shut my eyes. I needed to pray. I told Charles that I loved him and that I would call him later as if I were getting my hair done. We hung up and I prayed.

Gray World

When the machine started, and it did so with an intimidating loud hum. I turned the television up as loud as I could to drown it out. Exhaustion came upon me unlike nothing I felt in all the days of radiation treatment. Strength was being pulled right out of my body. Turned toward the oversized window at the grayish trees and prayed.

If their color was bright green, I would have felt alive, but they seemed gray and dull. Years of building a relationship with God became valued right now. I thanked

God for being with me when no one else could, and I prayed that it worked. I knew God was in the room with me. How? Because he said he would never leave me nor forsake me;

"Be strong and of good courage, fear not nor be afraid of them: for the Lord thy God, he it is that doth go with thee; he will not fail the nor forsake thee." (KJV), (Deuteronomy 31:6).

My system felt overloaded. Laying there, I recalled testimonies from people who were ill, and they stated 'I knew it all along. I just knew that God would to heal me', but that's not what I felt. I knew God could heal me and that it was God's will that I be healed but, as for His perfect will for my life, that I did not know. I was not be presumptuous.

Through all of this, I knew God's will was being done because this couldn't even touch my life if God did not permit it. I couldn't help but wonder if my time on this earth was up or not. What if I fulfilled my purpose already? I knew of other people who were devout Christians that died of illnesses. I was never presumptuous about God's will. All I knew was that I was on a journey I didn't have control over.

It was three o'clock in the morning and the machine was running. I awoke with a terrible pain in my abdomen. I remember calling the nurse and a few moments later the machine stopped. The doctor rushed in. His hair tussled, and a radiation badge swung from his neck.

They entered the room and looked at their radiation badges, then he passed a radiation wand over my body from my neck to my feet. He ordered an x-ray. In minutes, a technician came in and did the x-ray.

I prayed and wiped a few tears too. When they left, I called Charles. I didn't want to wake him up because I knew he had to be up in a few hours for work, but I needed to hear his voice and his prayers. Besides, he would be upset to learn that I didn't let him know what was going on.

The doctor's concern was that a radioactive implant shifted. After explaining, Charles prayed, and I told him to get some rest and I'd call him when the results were back. Minutes later, the doctor came in. This time he walked in with a relaxed expression. My nurse, whose face looked very concerned earlier, was now smiling.

"It's gas." He said relieved.

I think I blushed from embarrassment. The nurse held out an anti-gas chewable. It was a relief, and the anti-gas chewable worked fast. That was the only time I was glad that the door was shut and couldn't be opened. I called Charles and we laughed about it together. When everyone left the room, I lifted my hands and thanked God. Three days have never passed so slowly.

Leaving there felt wonderful. I will never forget what my nurse said to me as she wheeled me to my car.

"I hope I never see you again." She said with a smile.

I laughed and understood completely.

"I hope I never see you again either." We smiled and when the car door shut and I felt the cool leather seat beneath me, I was grateful.

The entire treatment was behind me and it felt so good to be home. So good to hold my children and hear their laughter. My dog greeted me excitedly and stayed by my side as usual. There was a new freshness in our home. Looking back, I gained a new appreciation for things I was around every day. Minor things I took for granted and even complained about.

Now I realized how valuable it was to just be able to do laundry at will. Prior, I didn't fully appreciate the blessing of being able to move and function without help. Through this circumstance, I felt a fresh appreciation for life and everything in it. Even everyday chores that I once dreaded seemed like a pleasure.

A fresh wind blew into my life. I was never a complainer or ungrateful at all, but looking back, there were times I neglected to praise, when I could have. Now, I couldn't wait to get back to my full strength so I could do all of those things again.

Home at Last

Home smelled great. That was the first thing that struck me. The hospital was stringent and antiseptic. It tired me. I felt drained. Charles helped me into bed immediately. Now, all we could do was wait for the results of the last battery of tests they took before I left the hospital.

Waking to the chatter of the children and the dog barking was like a dream come true. Sounds of home. Charles and I talked, made jokes and ate together. I felt lighter just knowing that the treatments were over. The next hurdle, waiting to find out if it worked.

I was so glad that treatment was over that I tried to get back to normalcy but found nothing was normal. There was a clock ticking in the back of my mind and the 'what if' thoughts were soaking in. They seemed ever looming and brought a heaviness with them. Also, my body functioned at a fraction of its true capability. I was weak and breathless.

One positive change was in my relationship with God. When I was ten years old, I got upset with my parents for moving us to a new house very far from where we were. I was sad because I had to leave my friends and like a child would, I saw nothing wrong with our house. However, my parents' view was vast. They saw the slight changes in our neighborhood that I couldn't see. They saw a better neighborhood with a great middle school and an award-winning high school. They saw an opportunity to put us somewhere better than where we were. Now, far more mature, I know that if they stayed in that neighborhood, I would have been a different person and my life may have taken a different path. They saw what I couldn't see and moved despite my feelings.

My consolation was that I trusted them. They did nothing for my demise. Now, in this, I established a deeper trust in God. Although I didn't like this 'move', this shift in my health, this scary circumstance, I trusted Him. He never did anything for my demise. He wants the best for me.

"For I know the thoughts that I think toward you, saith the Lord, thoughts of peace, and not of evil, to give you an expected end." (KJV) Jeremiah 29:11.

I prayed the healing scriptures, proclaimed and declared my healing, and whole-heartedly knew that God could heal me. Thus, the abundant scope of trust laid in the words 'I trust you Lord'.

Repeatedly, I thought about wanting to see my children grow up. Wanting to see them get married and one day hold my grandchildren. I wanted to grow old with Charles and take walks with him in far-off lands. We had so much left to explore and discover together.

Most of all, at the top of the list in importance was not wanting to put Charles through having to bury me and raise our children alone. I didn't want my parents to see a casket with their child in it. Those thoughts grayed my days even more than the cancer. I fought them. I prayed they lifted for a while. Then, the next day, the battle began again. I felt as if I was fighting mentally, spiritually and physically twenty-four hours a day.

There was no forgetting. The tiredness was perpetual and the change in our living routine was obvious. Charles carried far more than he should have had to, and I hated to think he may have to do this continuously if the results weren't favorable. There was nothing left to do except rest and wait.

Hope on the Other Side

CHAPTER SIX

Present Day...The Verdict

Seated on the sofa, I'm surrounded by more piles of clean, neatly folded laundry than any human being should have, I enjoyed every minute of folding. Soft clean blue jeans in every shade of blue. The afternoon sun is at full strength and I should draw the curtains but haven't gotten up the strength to stand again. My eyes are sensitive to the sun.

The laundry room is clean and empty, and there is nothing left for me to busy my hands with. Coffee, maybe I'll make some coffee. No, that may only make me more anxious. I don't want to call anyone. Talking to someone would be too much in my mind. There is enough going on up there as it is. Besides, I cannot hold a conversation without sounding breathless.

I left a message earlier with Tessa, the nurse. She knows me well and has always been very good about getting back to me, so I don't understand this delay. She told me that they usually give lab results in the morning. I tap the telephone beneath my hand. Lately, it's kept close in case of an emergency. The television is still playing one of my favorite church services. The oversized yellow tent glowed beneath a dark New York sky every night for six weeks in the summer. Folding chairs line up as pews with sawdust beneath them face the altar with a clear podium in the center.

Night after night we saw why God guided the pastor to come out of the air-conditioned sanctuary and set it up despite the expense. Drug dealers, prostitutes, drug addicts those who may not come to a church building were drawn by the Holy Spirit and stood in the outskirts leaning on trees listening to the service from a distance. By the end of the night, they were on the alter laying down guns, crack pipes and starting a new life in that sawdust.

I saw miracle after miracle first-hand. This service was exactly what I needed to see today. It played at least four times already, but I didn't care.

I need to go into my personal prayer closet. For the last six weeks, I held my breath now; I am ready to exhale. I walk into my prayer closet and close the door behind me. The carpet is warm beneath my feet. I know that I don't have the strength or breath to pray in words.

My prayers are silent, a murmur or tear. I turn my face toward heaven and tears stream down my cheeks. God hears tears. He understands our moans and groans. Faintly, I hear the video playing through the closed closet door. The closet is a large perfect square with clothes hung on three sides on double racks. Weakness overtakes me. I had pushed some clothes aside on the bottom rack weeks ago. I grip the bare wood bar.

"I just need to know what your will is." I mutter softly.

Then, I heard something that I have never heard before. The silence broke. This time, there was no still small voice. I heard God roar.

"NO MORE! NO MORE! THESE ENEMIES YE SHALL SEE NO MORE!"

I grab my head on either side, the words echo in my head. Down on my knees, the words swept through me like a wind from storm. A flood of deliverance sweeps over me.

A passion in His voice, like that of a parent unable to bear watching their child's suffering any longer. There was no room for mistake. No chance for me to wonder about what I heard. I open my eyes and immediately, lightness overtakes me. The weight of the diagnosis lifts off my shoulders.

One thing I know for certain, God always keeps His word. The only thing that can impede God fulfilling a promise to us, is us. I rest in His presence.

After some time, I step out of the closet and the air conditioner cools me immediately. Finally, I know the outcome. Finally, I know God's will for me. I smile inside because God has NEVER broken His word to me. Relieved, I call the doctor's office for my confirmation so that when Charles calls me on his lunch break, I will have good news for him.

"The doctor is not back yet, Janice. The results are here, I have them in my hand. I'll have her call as soon as she gets in." Says Tessa.

"Read it to me Tessa, please." I say happily.

I know what it's going to say, but my ears want to hear it. This is the testimony I have been waiting for since I got the diagnosis.

"I really am not supposed to... it's kind of technical and in numbers-"

"Please, it's okay, just tell me what you see."

My faith is high, and I stand straight up. Joyful anticipation is darting like electricity through me from my head to my feet. She reads then her words slide into being a mutter.

"What? Can you repeat that part?" I ask.

"I'm sorry. I'm not well versed in this, but I've seen many of these reports before. Janice, it doesn't look like it worked. I'm so sorry. I'll have the doctor call you, alright?" She says flatly.

No?

"Thank you, Tessa." I hang up the phone.

I'm confused. I know what I heard. There was no mistaking it. That wasn't 'me'. It was not wishful thinking. There was nothing to fiddle with. The laundry is done. Breathless, I walk into the family room and the church's tent service is at the end.

The words that the doctor spoke to me about quality of life if the treatment didn't work plays in my head. I wish they didn't. I wish I didn't remember them in such detail. She said that the procedure's result is given as a score. If the score is between within a certain range, it didn't work which means the cancer is likely to return and in doing so, it would spread quickly. Her recommendation at that point would be total exoneration, which is the removal of organs from my urinary, gastrointestinal and gynecologic systems. A part of the large intestine (colon), rectum and anus would be removed. Removal of the end of the large would require me to have a colostomy. Going to the bathroom would change for me for the rest of my life.

My ovaries, fallopian tubes, and uterus would be removed meaning that I couldn't have any more children. Life as I know it would change not only for myself but for Charles and our children. I would require dialysis for the rest of my life. Even with all of this, it was likely that the cancer would return.

This situation gives additional weight to the term, 'God willing'. Finally, I surrendered ALL. I surrendered my will completely. A wave of certainty flows over me in the peace that met me in the prayer closet. I know what I heard in my prayer closet, but it doesn't stop the storm that is trying to rage in my mind. The difference is that the results no longer matter. My mind is made up.

The choir is sings, "I Surrender All". I take a deep breath and lift my hands as high as I can and wave them back and forward slowly. In my heart, I accept God's will for my life, regardless of what it may be. I decide, whatever my fate, the God of Abraham, Isaac, and Jacob, is *my* God until my end and I will serve Him until my last breath.

I praise God, lifting one foot at a time in a slow stepping motion with my hands lifted. I mouth the words to the song, too breathless to sing. Tears stream down my face because whatever my end, I will worship until... the end.

"I worship you. You are my God. You're still my God. I'll worship you and serve you all the days of my life." Lifting one foot at a time in a slow methodical marching motion for as long as I can, I praise. "I give you all I can, right now!"

I open my eyes and the video has stopped playing. I wash my face. The cold water feels good. I don't recognize the person in the mirror. She's not the carefree woman I once knew. She's changed somehow. Yes, her eyes are swollen, and nose is red, but that's not what has changed. She's connected in a deeper way to her best friend, who never left her side.

He was there in the doctor's office when they first told her she had cancer. He was there in the car while driving to M. D. Anderson. He was in the room when the enormous doors shut, and the machine started. He's here right now.

This woman is accepting of the things she can't control and willing to fight to change the things she can control. She's more than grateful. Gentle yet, relentless. She's more than what she was before the diagnosis. I like her.

I walk to the family room curtains, grasp them high on either side to close them to block the scorching Houston sun, then, I pause. The sun on my face, I shut my eyes, letting it warm me. I'm alive and it's a beautiful day. Things aren't what they used to be, but I'm still here. The colors are still muted but I can see them. A calm settles on me. My mind is still, and I feel my friend right here with me. Here, alone in the house. I know that I am not by myself. The phone rings. It must be Charles. I take a breath.

"Praise the Lord." I say.

I expected to hear Charles's voice, but it isn't him.

"Janice!" A voice says frantically.

My heart leaps. It is the doctor.

"Yes, Dr. Thomas?" I stammer.

I walk into the bedroom and sit on the foot of the bed. She probably learned that I know the results and will tell me the next steps. My hand is trembling slightly, and I catch my breath while she speaks.

"I was hoping I caught you," she says. I hear papers rustle. "Tessa was wrong, Janice. She was wrong! Janice, it worked! You're clear."

"WHAT! Wait," my trembling hand covers my mouth loosely. "… please hold on, I need to... I have to get Charles on the line!"

"Go ahead." she says happily.

He answered his phone immediately.

"Babe!" I blurt, "Dr. Thomas is on the line. She has the results! I will put you into the call."

"All right, yes." He says.

I can barely find the button on the phone. Everything is blurry through my tears.

"Dr. Thomas, we're here. Go ahead." I say.

"It worked guys! It worked. Not only did it work, success is presumed if you score between a five and eight. The lower the number, the better. You are zero!"

"What!" My Darling yells.

"Thank you, God!" we yell simultaneously.

"I'll send you this report. Congratulations, guys. Janice, I hope I never see you again. Goodbye." She laughs as she hangs up.

I understand. I laugh for joy and drop to my knees beside the bed.

"Babe, I'll call you back. I need to go, thank God." I say.

"Me too!" Says Charles.

I hang up the phone, lift my head and see the prayer closet door in front of me. I stand slowly and walk toward it. I put my hand on the doorknob. The doorknob I grabbed so many times since this journey started. I open it and step inside. With all my strength, I lift my hands, tilt my face toward heaven and praise.

"Lord I thank you. Thank you, God! Hallelujah!" I repeat in a whisper until I'm just moving my lips.

And He speaks.

"I like this praise. But I like the other one better. The one you gave me when it looked like I did not do what I said I would do."

I drop to my knees and smile, shaking my head. I understand.

Hope on the Other Side

CHAPTER SEVEN

Beautiful

- [ ] Grocery Shop
- [ ] Bike Ride Date
- [ ] Laundry
- [ ] Cook Dinner
- [ ] Wash Dog
- [ ] Break Garden Ground

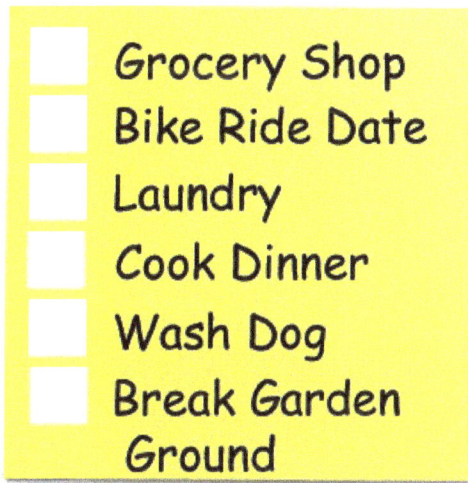

I walk to the family room and look out of the window and see the most beautiful view. The colors are back. Green is green and yellow is yellow. My heart beats with gratitude. The trees burst with color and a small patch of lavender flowers just beneath them sway slightly in the hot breeze.

There is a road to recovery, and this is my first step. I have a grateful mind. My body will catch up. It has no choice. Something brushes against my ankle. I look down to my right and there is my faithful fluffy friend. His name, Praise. Fitting, especially right now. He sits beside me and looks up at me. Even he looks relieved.

Charles comes home with a dinner in hand and we had the best celebration ever. I don't want to sleep. Every moment of life is fresh. There is no shadow over my head or looming fears. My body is still weak, and the recovery road is long, but I will keep every follow-up appointment, eat healthy and listen to my body.

My usual to-do list has returned. I smiled when I wrote the last item. I will plant my garden and live to watch it grow. The conception of the baby was the catalyst that got me to the doctor's office. I was so busy making business plans and getting things laid out for this next phase of our life that going to the doctor for check-ups was not on my to-do list. I know now that if it were not for the pregnancy, the cancer would not have been found. There were no symptoms. Nothing.

Looking back, we didn't know why God gave us the unction to move to Houston Texas. We didn't know we would need M. D. Anderson. We didn't know that it was rated the best cancer center in the world or that my radiologist was well known for giving seminars all over the world. She teaches other radiologists to do the procedure that she did on me.

My Life After Surviving A Diagnosis

Overall, there was a lot we did not know. But God knew. God was guiding us when we didn't even know it. At my first follow-up appointment my doctor looked at my medical chart then double checked the date of my treatment. I didn't know why until after the examination.

"Is everything all right?" I ask her.

"Yes. Absolutely, it's just that... well, according to the treatment date in your chart, your treatment was four months ago." She says pointing to her tablet.

"That's correct." I confirm.

"But your body is showing over six months of healing. I don't know what you're doing but keep doing it. Your skin looks great and you have no signs of the typical after-effects of that treatment." She gazes at me.

I smile because this was the moment that a person usually takes the credit by thanking the person for their compliment and attributing it to good eating or rest etcetera. For me, I knew this was the moment I had to give honor to whom honor is due.

"To God be the glory." I said smiling widely.

I am still humbled each time I walk into that facility for my follow-up visit. It reminds me of my mortality. To this day, I think it would be a good idea for people to visit any cancer facility. I never saw myself as a complainer because I am grateful for the here and now. Yet, after my M. D.

Anderson experience, I smile when I clean out the fridge and do the everyday mundane things that just have to get done.

Oh, and that business plan, well, it wasn't forgotten. That's another testimony but, I'll give you a hint. With God's guidance and favor, we started a Wholesale and logistics company whose products were on the shelves of over eighty-five Kroger grocery stores. The largest grocery store chain in the United States.

The road of treatment is a road with bumps and dips, but one that God can see you through if you let Him. Perhaps you are reading this and your loved one is on the examination table. You both can survive a diagnosis. Be kind, be patient and stay encouraged because there is hope on the other side.

Keys to Surviving A Diagnosis

The Approach

An airplane will circle the airways until it is properly aligned for its landing. When all circumstances are in order, it will safely land on the runway. Your approach to your health should be optimistic and realistic. Go for examinations and do not allow fear to keep you from seeking medical attention. Early intervention is key in most medical conditions. The sooner things are addressed, the better. Use the faith scriptures in The Workbook to get you into the right frame of mind to face the possibilities of a diagnosis with strength and believe God for healing. Thus, you will approach your health from an optimistic and faith-filled angle.

The Touch Down

Landing gear is the mechanism in an airplane specifically created for the airplanes landing. They design it to bear the weight of the airplane and enable it to be mobile on the surface of the earth. They do not need landing gear when the plane is flying. Then it is tucked safely away while the airplane soars.

Like landing gear, your faith is something that should always be present with you. It must be strong to bear whatever comes your way. When it is needed, you pull it out and use it. Faith, like the tire on the landing gear, cushions the blow for you when you leave one atmosphere (completely healthy with an excellent report) and enter another (diagnosed with an illness). It eases you into the transition and allows you to move as necessary in your new plain.

Does this mean you accept your diagnosis as being permanent? No. Accepting a diagnosis and taking your physician's medical advice does not mean that you must accept your condition as permanent. You see, landing gear works two ways. It assists the plane when landing and when taking off.

Believe whole-heartedly that it is God's plan for your life to recover. Use the same faith to believe and know that God wants the best for you and that His thoughts toward you are good and not evil. Janice understood this, and her faith enabled her to believe until the end. She was prepared to hold on to her belief in God regardless of what her outcome was.

Disembark

Your faith has taken you through facing your worst fear, you have landed in your new reality now, disembark and begin the new journey. Take a deep breath and step into it. The aircraft has done its job. Now, you simply have to continue in faith and use the tools in the "Surviving A Diagnosis, Hope on the Other Side & The Workbook" to walk through your journey.

It may feel like a strange land. An unfamiliar place that you are uncertain how to navigate through. You may not be intended to stay in this unknown land. Like Janice, this may be your first encounter with a medical condition. Asking questions is a significant start. Additional tips to use are in the Workbook. You can take it to your doctor's office as it is a log of your daily medical stats. Feed your faith with the podcast designed and online course. Don't lose hope on the other side.

SNEAK PEAK OF THE WORKBOOK

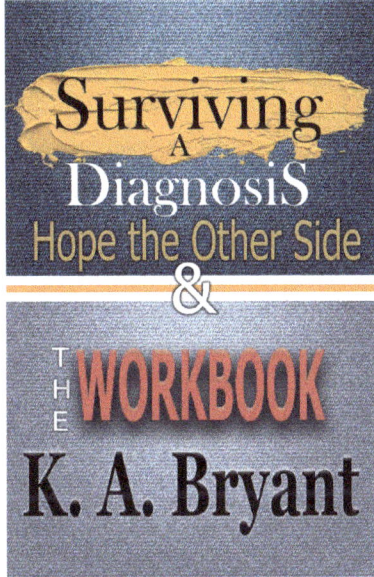

Introduction

Grab a pen or pencil and let's get into it. This workbook is laid out with easy-to-read titles and subtitles so you can navigate back to the pages you want to go to with ease.

To get in-dept teaching and inspirational information in audio and video format, there is an online course and podcast available. See more on kabryant.com.

Stay in touch by joining the mailing list. Reading is a great way to pass the time. I was touched by a story of a man who read books during his chemotherapy treatment because it helped him to take his mind off of his unpleasant procedure. Because of this, I put a sample of the first book of the fiction series at the back of the book.

This workbook is interactive and challenges your thinking about your mind, body, and spirit.

Thank you for choosing this book.

Mind

It would be a misconception to think a physical illness only affects someone physically. The impact of an illness whether it be an injury or a terminal diagnosis spans beyond the affected area. Post-traumatic Stress Disorder (P. T. S. D.) is evidence of that. The after effect of a traumatic experience can linger long after the experience is over. The same is true for an illness.

Have you ever met anyone who said that they were afraid of getting an illness because one of their parents or grandparents had it? They may have never had a symptom yet, the fear of it manifesting in their lives is enough for them to carry a feeling of dread in the back of their mind. Is it an illogical fear?

Perhaps not. However, just because it is logical to be fearful doesn't mean you have to remain in fear.

"And the peace of God, which passeth all understanding, shall keep your hearts and minds through Christ Jesus." (KJV), Philippians 4:7.

The feeling of fear tries to come to all of us as human beings, at some time. However, it doesn't mean we have to let it stay and build a home in our minds. Once fear moves in it brings in the "What if's".

What if I lose my job? What if I get sick? What if I can't pay the taxes? What if my parent dies? What if my business fails? The list can go on and on. Fear is the core reason many people can't sleep at night and wake with anxiety and ultimately carry an extensive amount of stress daily. Stress can trigger high blood pressure and other medically related things in our bodies. So how do we turn off the faucet of fear? The answer is to use of the countermeasure to fear. What is the countermeasure of fear? Faith.

Definition of Body by Merriam Webster:

faith noun

    2 b (1): firm belief in something for which there is no proof

There are a few definitions for faith, but this one is the one we will use for this purpose. There is no proof that you will never lose your job. There is no proof that you will not get the illness that your mother or father had. There is no proof that your business will survive an economic hardship yet there is faith. (continues)

PG. 110_____

Medical Contact

My Team

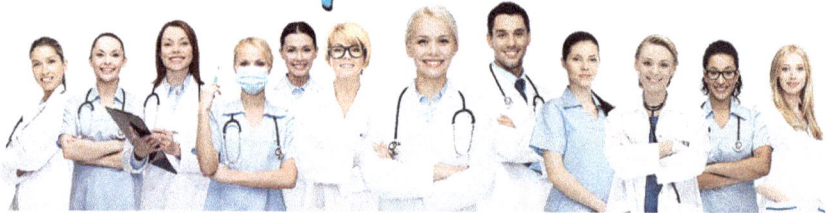

There is a team of people assigned to your care. From the receptionist that schedules your appointments to your doctor. It is easy to overlook some parts of your care team, but all of them are significant to your health plan. Thank the medical assistant or nurse that leads you to your examination

Keep reading...

"Surviving A Diagnosis, Hope on the Other Side &

The Workbook" (2 books in 1).

The book contains this book and the workbook.

Available in Paperback.

Scriptures

Scriptures are quoted from the King James version of the Bible.

Mark 9:23... "Jesus said unto him, If thou canst believe, all things are possible to him that believeth."

Luke 8:50... "But when Jesus heard it, he answered him, saying Fear not: believe only, and she shall be made whole."

Psalm 147:3... "He health the broken in heart, and bindeth up their wounds."

Mark 10:52... "And Jesus said unto him, Go thy way; thy faith hath made thee whole. And immediately he received his sight, and followed Jesus in the way."

James 5:14-15... "Is any sick among you? Let him call for the elders of the church; and let them pray over

him, anointing him with oil in the name of the Lord: And the prayer of faith shall save the sick, and the Lord shall raise him up; and if he have committed sins, they shall be forgiven him.
James 5:16... "Confess your faults to one another, and pray one for another that ye may be healed. The effectual fervent prayer of a righteous man availeth much.

Proverbs 17:22... "A merry heart doeth good like a medicine: but a broken spirit drieth the bones.

2 Chronicles 7:14... "If my people which are called by my name shall humble themselves, and pray, and seek my face, and turn from their wicked ways; then will I hear from heaven, and will forgive their sin, and will heal their land.

1 Peter 2:24... "Who his own self bare our sins in his own body on the tree, that we, being dead to sins should live unto righteousness: by whose stripes ye were healed.

Hope on the Other Side

BEYOND THE BOOK

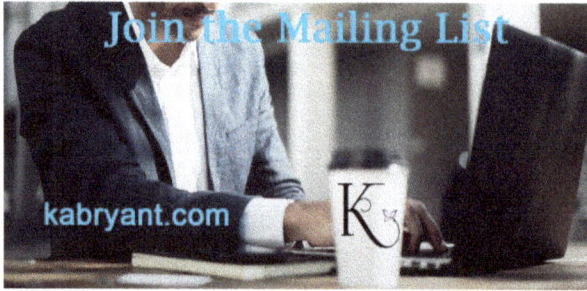

Get new release deals, free books, and any promotional give-aways coming up. I respect your email box and only send things I feel you want to know about.

What you'll get...

Monthly Newsletter Book Promotions Pre-Release Offers New Book Release Deals & Give-aways. Type the link below into your

browser:

https://www.kabryant.com/join-

mailer Join free with one click.

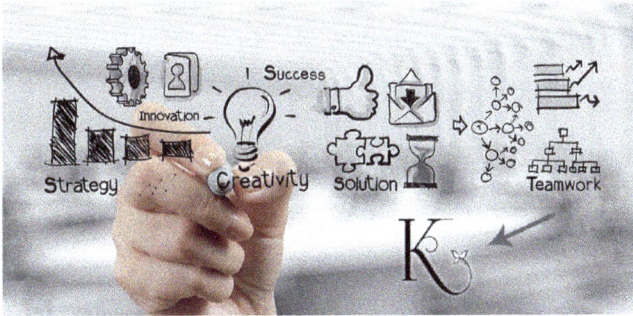

Online Courses & Podcast

World events have caused many people to take on additional roles. The online courses and podcast, K-Today, delivers the content you need. A monthly newsletter and blog are delivered to your email box. Live Your Life With Kay delivers solutions for success. It guides you to find the strategy to unlock your creativity.

Work at your own pace and review the areas you want to focus on. Priceless, for the peace of mind it will bring. Also, I will teach you how to homeschool using the supplies you already have at home. If you want to go-pro and purchase items, I tell you what to get and how to use it.

Get your online course on the K.A. Bryant's official

Websites

Liveyourlifewithkay.com and

kabryant.com/ktoday

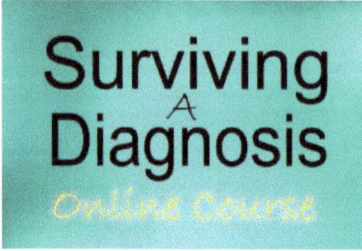

Extension of the Surviving A Diagnosis book. It details helpful tips and builds your faith.

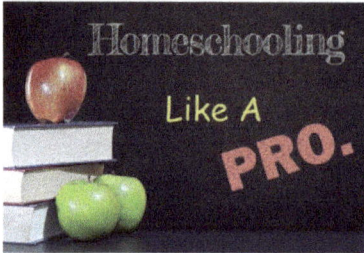

Parents have become teacher/caretaker while juggling work as well. You don't have to feel your way through it. I took over a decade of teaching and management experience and put it into this course using audio and video features.

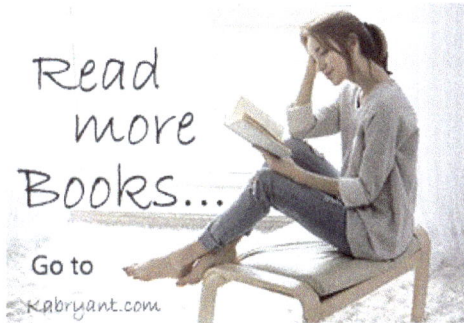

Read more Books...

Go to kabryant.com

Jumping into that other world priceless. Hot cup in hand, I started writing for the love of writing and can't think of anything I would rather do for the rest of my life. Once a writer, always a writer. A vision grew to draw a leisure reader, confined patient, or a child on summer vacation with their feet twirling in the grass, into a new world between two covers. I want to invite you to join the mailing list to stay informed of all the new upcoming promotions and book give-away.

Type the link in your browser:

https://www.kabryant.com/copy-of-books

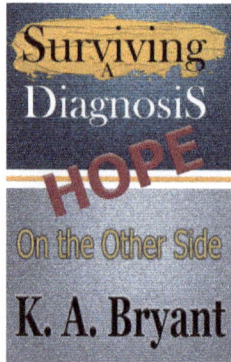

Non-Fiction, True account, inspirational, informative

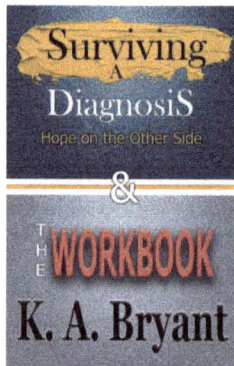

Non-Fiction, True account, inspirational, informative with fillable charts and logs.

Description:
      Two books in one. "Hope on the Other Side"
      with "The Workbook".

Perfect for a patient or caregiver. Designed as a useful tool for someone facing a long-term illness, long-term care, or short-term care. An inspirational thread is woven into the fabric of the book with its roots based in Christianity.

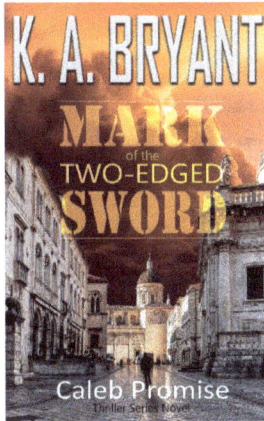

Fiction Espionage, Thriller-Mystery, Easy Reading, Page-turner

Description:
Caleb Promise Series Mission 1

First book in the Caleb Promise Series, Mission One. A deep 627 Page meaty thriller, espionage, and political mystery novel. There is a dystopian thread through the book with a literary hand. Bursts with suspense, emotional rides, and espionage at the highest levels of government.

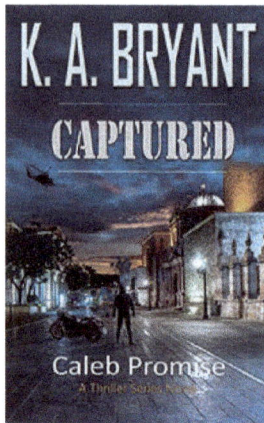

Fiction Espionage, Thriller-Mystery, Easy Reading, Page-turner

Description:
Caleb Promise Series Mission 2

An attack on United States soil can't go unanswered. One captured man's rescue could prevent war, but only if Caleb Promise denies his instincts. A government coup is in flow. His orders, to extract the CAPTURED man but leave the man's wife, Tempest Bleu. The problem is, he can't.

After his mission in <u>Mark of the Two- Edged Sword</u>, Caleb finally feels a settling come into his life. He can't rest yet. Pulled into finding the CAPTURED man, Caleb evolves. In mission one, he peeks his head into the shadowed life of an undercover agent.

However, now, in CAPTURED he is sanguine. This is the life for him. He moves into his calling sure-footed thus more adept. He realizes his values as an agent is being defined in this mission and his journey has just begun.

FOR READERS, BLOGGERS, POD-CASTERS, YOU-TUBERS AND BOOK REVIEWERS

SPECIAL OFFER:

Reviews are a tremendous influence online, and it would really help me reach my writing goal if you would write a quick review. Your feedback tells me what you want to see more or less of.

I can write it, but I need you to push it. If you are a Blogger, Pod-Castor, You-Tuber or Book Reviewer, I invite you to join the street team. A vetted influencer can get pre-launch peeks at books.

I believe we never stop learning. It's a lifelong gift to grow and change.

Type the link in your bowser:

Https://www. kabryant.com/street-team-sign-up

Hope on the Other Side

K

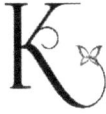

K.A. BRYANT, Author

Letter from the author

I still remember how warm it was in Mrs. Harris's English class. She liked it that way although she wore a sweater. I don't know why I was always distracted by her long bead necklaces she pulled on habitually. That was when teachers wore silk blouses, long skirts down to their mid-calf with stockings and shoes that clicked when they walked.

She was a retired play-write with her passion for the written word evident in her detailed critique of every short story scrawled by the twenty children in the class. She was the catalyst. The pointed finger saying, 'go that way'. All I knew was it was fun. Oh, the simple thinking era.

Life, time, and the Internet soon showed me that there was so much more to writing. The wonderful thing was discovering a world of wonderful people with either a love of reading, writing, or both so willing to share their opinions and be a pointed finger.

Much time has passed since Mrs. Harris's class, but I'm still going in the direction of that pointed finger.

My hope... is that my journey in writing will find my books in the hands of readers all over the world and inspire someone to reach further, write more, or just explore their dream. Hope can be lost when you are going through a long, seemingly endless difficult time, just as the main character Caleb Promise experienced. In the book, keeping focused on his mission pulled him out of the pit-experience he was in. An experience that was draining him of his strength and willingness to live.

You and I... can propel a vision beyond expectation by taking three easy steps:

1. Sign-up to stay informed.
2. Write a review online after reading a book.
3. Tell your friends.

You can stay in touch with me by Twitter @kabryantauthor, Facebook @kabryantbooks. I am also on Instagram, GoodReads and WordPress. If you enjoy the books and blogs, you can show your support on Patreon.com.

Thank you for reading the book!

SNEAK PEAK OF A BOOK

Hope on the Other Side

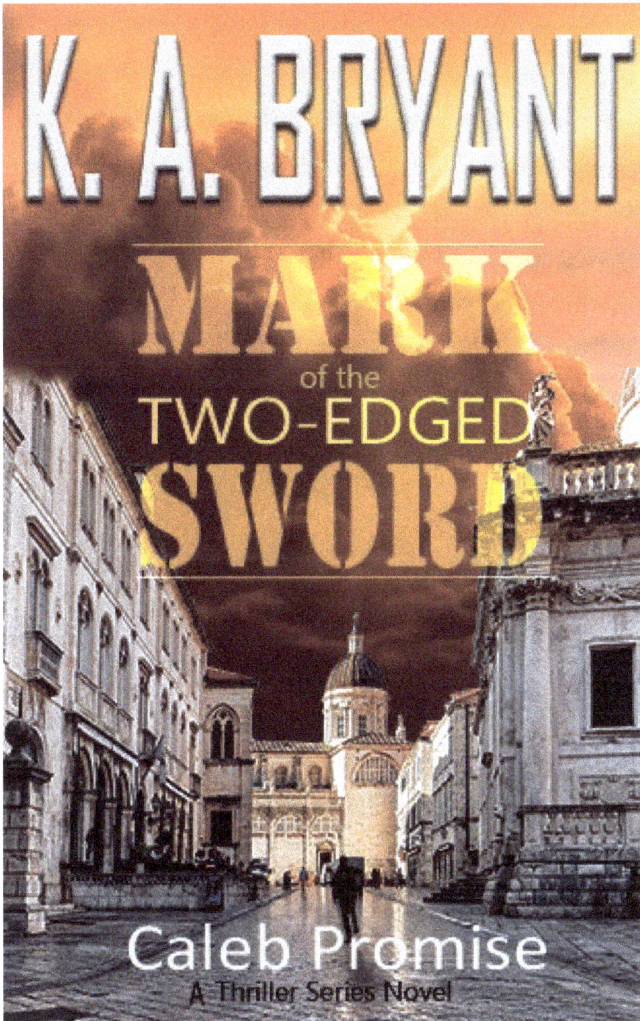

Hope on the Other Side

CHAPTER ONE

CALEB PROMISE

The tree isn't wide enough, not nearly wide enough. It never is. Being a man that is six foot two inches, isn't helping. My broad shoulders are sticking out. I can feel it. It will see me. Maybe if I crouch. It isn't finished yet. Not even close. The sound of my heart pounding seems louder than their screams, and it hears everything. That's how it found them underground in that muddy tunnel covered by the fall leaves.

They hid for weeks. A group here, a group there. Don't ask me how I know, I just do. Thin, rationing food for months. I can hear them praying as it holds them up like trophies in front of the government vehicle's lights. The agents, bored now, slump in their seats. The cold frost of their breath glows in the headlights.
Taller than any human, the face of a lioness and arms of a gorilla. That's all I ever see. It fades into shadows. No matter how hard I try, I never see all of it. Why am I always barefoot?
People who don't have this think it's cool, but it's not. Consciousness in a dream used to be fun. The ability to choose

which way to go, whether to fly or walk and even to wake up or not. It's not fun. I don't truly rest. Ever. Especially in this dream. It has returned every night for weeks.

I must get to that rock without it hearing me. From there, I may see it. All of it. There she is. The lady with the red hair. The creature turns around right after pulling her out. This is my chance.
I take one step. It's over. I felt it crack beneath my foot. My eyes close, praying it didn't hear me. But I know it did. I open my eyes. It's staring right at me.

It opens its claw, releasing her. It's coming. The ground vibrates with each step. I can't hear anything except my heart pounding. She's falling to the ground, but the drop encompasses me.
I jolt awake. Sitting straight up. My room is as cold and clammy as the dream. It's over, but the eeriness of the dream hangs in the air with the feeling that someone else was in that forest. Someone watches with a disconnected heart. Alive enough, but uncaring. Unaffected by what they saw.

A shiver runs up my back. The cheap flat coverlet in my grip lost its usefulness months ago. Now it only keeps the roaches from falling on my sheets. I had no choice. This is where the orphanage arranged for me to live after I turned eighteen. It has been three years now living in this hotel-style living quarter. Wow, it seems as if I've been here much longer than that. I feel older than that. I don't want to get up yet.

I give in, flop back onto the flat dingy pillow and draw the cover up to my chin. My full beard and hair soaked from perspiration. The rubber band I used to tie my hair back for work last night is now poking me in the ear.

It won't be long now. The shivering has begun and even with my eyes closed, the room spins violently, and my head is pulsing.

"Shut up!" I yell.

The neighbors on the other side of the thin wall are always fighting. Every morning a blaring argument with their morning coffee about why he came home so late.

"You shut up!" She yells back with two bangs on the wall, making the cheap framed photo above my head jump.

The pulsing turns into a full- blown blinding headache. I have to get up. I don't want to, but I have no choice. There it is, the chalky aspirin in the back of the night table drawer, right beside my keys and an unopened Gideon Bible. Flat soda works just at well, washing it down as a glass of cold water. I stagger into the bathroom. Funny, there's no heat, but the hot water in the shower works perfectly.

One advantage to being taller than average, I can reach the loose screws to the rusted vent in the wall easily. My hiding place. My fingers fumble around in the vent, searching for it. There it is. The dusty black sock guarding my life savings. The knot is smaller than last month. It started shrinking when my dream started shrinking. I can't help but give it a squeeze right before I put it away, a mental measurement of how much I have to put back if I ever regain hope of getting out of here. Where is the key? There, inside a fold in the sock, I feel it.

A small gold-tone key. I rub its outline between my fingers. It is a lifeline to reality. I have a feeling I'll be needing it soon. I started saving money the week I began work. I started work the day after the orphanage driver dropped me at the front door, a wide-eyed country boy gazing at skyscrapers.

Manhattan is full of lavish apartments with doormen tipping their hats as residents walk in swinging shiny shopping bags. Fresh out of the orphanage, I honestly believed that could be me one day swinging those bags.

Hope. A gift from my parents. They always told me I could do and be anything. They told me I was smart and like any kid; I believed what my parents said. I never imagined the best I could be was the one holding the door. They never got to finish me. It's not their fault.

I can still remember the dress my mother wore to my fifteenth birthday party just three days before she and my father were killed in the accident. At least then, I thought it was an accident. I can't think about that right now.

Housekeeping is coming today. Nothing spurs change like three police raids and a threat to be shut down. They knock on the door like the police. Hard and loud. When I open the door, if she suspects nothing, she hands me clean sheets and towels. If it's tied, she'll take the trash.

However, if she has any suspicions, she does a thorough 'cleaning' of the room. I noticed a pattern. These were no petite housekeepers wearing uniform dresses and nursing shoes. They always wore jeans and were more muscular than most men, with a pistol bulging in the small of their back.

The press-board dresser with sharp corners holds the residue of every meal I ate for the week. I can hear the three knocks of the housekeeper getting louder as she comes up the hall. I fold the pizza boxes and deli bags into the garbage can.

In the can's bottom, my empty bottles. They clank in the can, telling my life's story. The faster I move, the more the torn linoleum snags the bottom of my socks. I can't help but look at the crack in the corner of the large rectangular dresser mirror. It's not supposed to be there, maybe that's why it keeps catching my eye. It's the flaw in perfection. I thought of covering it, but it's got a right to be there, just like the rest of the mirror.

I'm tired. At twenty-one, I'm tired. Tired of being the crack in the mirror. I've been mistaken for being in my forties. Tiredness makes you look old and feel old.

A flash of light outside of my window draws my attention. The 'C' outside of my window was the first one in neon 'Vacancy' sign running vertically down the building and it is lit. It wasn't lit yesterday. She's here. Three loud bangs.

"Housekeeping."

I knot the top of the full garbage bag, drop it on the floor beside the door, and open the door. Bare-face, she looks at me emotionless. I snatch the sheets off of the bed into a ball and hold them out to her. She looks past me into the room. She isn't taken aback by my lean undershirt-clad physique.

She pushes past me, glances into the bathroom then drops the stack of clean sheets with towels on the bed. With gloved hands, she grabs the sheets from my hands and her cold stare reflects just how much she loves her job. One foot in the hall, she drops the sheets into the cart and grabs the garbage bag and walks out, leaving the door open behind her. A real ray of sunshine.

I look down at myself, sort of wondering why she wasn't in awe. I have a crease in my pants and everything. The cleaner's crease is always stiff, and the pant bottoms are wide enough to go over my black boots. I walk to the door to close it.

Out of habit, I look left and right down the hall before closing the door. She pushes the over-sized cart to the next room. My sarcasm gets the best of me., it's almost been a full five hours.

"And a Merry Christmas to you." I say.

As expected, she ignores me, rolling to the next room, but she pauses, she looks toward the floor to her left. What's over there? The cart passes revealing the hall prostitute with eyes dripping in makeup, knees drawn into her chest and back pressed to the wall of her pimp's apartment. A labored exhale.

I fell prey to her once. Not the way most would. One glance at those glazed eyes, bleach blond hair and it all came back. My ignorance. She's about my age. I felt bad for her. That night, the hall was dark, hot and smelly and I still had my streak of naivete fresh off the farm. I invited her in, offered her hot pizza and a cool breeze under my oscillating fan for the night. I gave her the bed and slept on the floor.

I woke to a boot in my gut and watched her willingly obey her large under dressed pimp to rob me of my last forty-five dollars. I know why she did it.   It wasn't for the obvious reason. I look at it as payment for what she brought with her.

Keep   reading...

Get   <u>Mark   of   the   Two-Edged Sword</u>

<u>Available where books are sold.</u>

Type   into   your   browser: kabryant.com

Sign up for the mailing list on:

Non-fiction:
Liveyourlifewithkay.com
https://www.liveyourlifewithkay.com

Fiction Books:
https://www.kabryant.com

www.ingramcontent.com/pod-product-compliance
Lightning Source LLC
Chambersburg PA
CBHW041929260326
41914CB00009B/1239